Dorsaf Aloui
Meriam Bouchekoua
Sonia Trabelsi

Imported malaria: Evaluation of 2 rapid diagnostic tests

Dorsaf Aloui
Meriam Bouchekoua
Sonia Trabelsi

Imported malaria: Evaluation of 2 rapid diagnostic tests

Performance of "ABON™ Plus Malaria®" and "iTest Malaria®" rapid tests in diagnosing imported malaria

ScienciaScripts

Imprint

Cover image: www.ingimage.com

This book is a translation from the original published under ISBN 978-613-8-49361-7.

Publisher:
Sciencia Scripts
is a trademark of
Dodo Books Indian Ocean Ltd. and OmniScriptum S.R.L publishing group

120 High Road, East Finchley, London, N2 9ED, United Kingdom
Str. Armeneasca 28/1, office 1, Chisinau MD-2012, Republic of Moldova, Europe
Printed at: see last page
ISBN: 978-620-8-26667-7

TABLE OF CONTENTS

INTRODUCTION

Malaria is a parasitic disease caused by haematozoa of the genus Plasmodium (P.), transmitted to humans by the bite of an insect vector, the female Anopheles [1]. It is the world's leading parasitic endemic, exposing almost half the world's population to the risk of contracting the disease [2].

According to the World Health Organisation (WHO), there will be 249 million cases and 608,000 deaths by 2022, 80% of which will be in children under the age of 5. This morbidity and mortality is exacerbated by the emergence and spread of chemo-resistant strains [2].

In Tunisia, malaria was endemo-epidemic, with an average incidence of around 10,000 cases per year [3]. Thanks to the national malaria eradication programme and, in particular, the various malaria control campaigns, especially those carried out between 1968 and 1972 with the help of the WHO, our country has seen an end to active transmission of this parasite since 1979, when the last indigenous case occurred [3,4]. Since then, only imported cases have been recorded, the incidence of which is on the increase due to the multiplicity of tourist, professional, commercial and humanitarian exchanges with malaria zones, as well as the increase in the number of students from endemic countries [5,6].

Thus, our country remains exposed to the risk of reintroduction of malaria because of the persistence of anophelism and the presence of these imported cases [4]. This calls for increased vigilance against the disease. In Tunisia, a country that has been in the prevention phase since 1996, the main strategies and policies of the current programme to prevent the re-emergence of malaria are epidemiological and entomological surveillance, rapid treatment of imported cases and prevention of transmission, one of the main activities of which is active screening and treatment of students who are not permanent residents of

Tunisia (ENRPT) [5]. The diagnosis of malaria is essentially parasitological. According to the WHO, the blood smear (FS) and the thick blood drop (GE) remain the reference techniques in terms of sensitivity and specificity, and should be used as the first line of defence. However, the reliability of these tests requires high-quality equipment (microscope) and qualified, experienced staff. For all these reasons, immunochromatographic rapid diagnostic tests (RDTs) have been developed to detect parasitic antigens in blood. Currently used in conjunction with microscopy, they have the advantage of being quick and easy to use, making it possible to orientate the diagnosis and speed up treatment. The aim of our work is to evaluate the performance of two rapid diagnostic tests ABON™ Plus Malaria® and iTest Malaria® compared with reference microscopic techniques, in the diagnosis of imported malaria in travellers to endemic areas and in screening non-permanent resident students in Tunisia (ENRPT).

METHODS

I. Presentation of the study

This was a descriptive retrospective study of all malaria cases collected in the Parasitology-Mycology laboratory of the Charles Nicolle Hospital in Tunis (HCN) over a period of three academic years: 2020-2021, 2021-2022 and 2022-2023.

II. Population study

- **Inclusion criteria :**

The study included :

- All cases of imported malaria diagnosed during the study period in Tunisian and foreign subjects referred to the Parasitology-Mycology laboratory of the Charles Nicolle Hospital in Tunis for suspected malaria (symptomatic subjects).

- Students not permanently resident in Tunisia (ENRPT) from malaria-infected countries who have been diagnosed as part of systematic screening. They were referred to the Parasitology-Mycology Laboratory by the Department of School and University Medicine as part of the national surveillance programme for this population.

- **Non-inclusion criteria :**

Subjects suspected of having malaria but in whom parasitological examination has not revealed Plasmodium sp.

III. Methods

1. Collection of data

For each patient or student, a pre-established information sheet has been drawn up. was completed on epidemiological, clinical and biological data.

2. Diagnosis parasitology

Plasmodium sp was tested directly. Each patient receivedd':

- A thick drop (GE),

- A blood smear (FS),

- One or two rapid diagnostic tests (RDTs) depending on availability

2.1. Direct debit

Blood samples were taken by venipuncture using an EDTA (ethylene diamine tetra acetic) tube. The samples were processed rapidly to avoid alteration of the parasites.

2.2. Drop thick

This is a concentration technique used to examine a large volume of blood in a small area. The GE is prepared by placing a drop of blood (2 to 5 µL) in the middle of the slide. It is then spread over a surface area of 1 cm² using the tip of another slide and circular defibrinating movements. The slide is then left to dry in a 37° oven. °C for 5 minutes (emergency) or in ambient air.

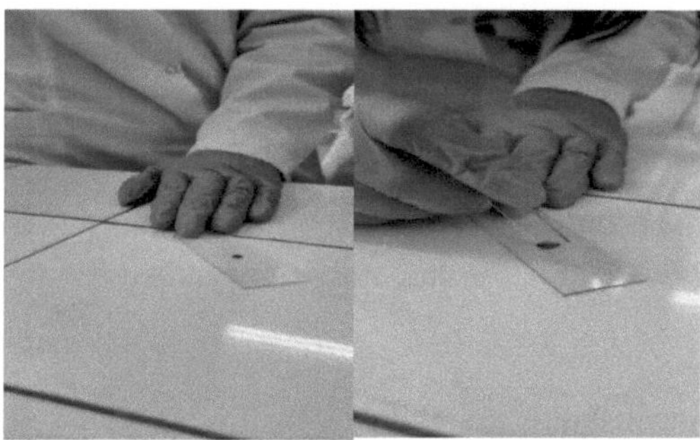

Figure 1: Making a thick drop

(HCN Parasitology Laboratory)

Giemsa staining was used and microscopic observation was carried out at X1000 magnification using immersion oil, exploring a minimum of 100 fields. The Giemsa solution stains the cytoplasm of the plasmodia blue and the chromatin intense red. EW has the advantage of being a more sensitive technique, making up for the false negatives of FS. However, it cannot be used to diagnose the plasmodium species and requires considerable experience on the part of the observer.

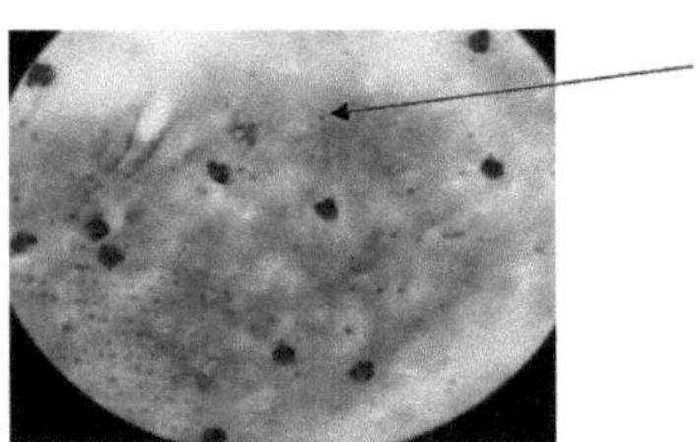

Figure 2: Trophozoites of Plasmodium sp on GE (Giemsa stain/obj x 100/ HCN parasitology laboratory)

2.3. Blood smear

This involves spreading a quantity of whole blood in a thin layer over an object blade. It consists of :

-Place a drop of blood of approximately 2µl on the end of a slide.

-Place a second blade at a 45° angle in contact with the drop of blood so that it spreads by capillary action along the edge of the blade.

-Slide the blade forward quickly, smoothly and evenly, maintaining the same angle.

-A good quality smear should end with a clear fringed area.

-Dry quickly to avoid shrinkage of leukocytes and deformation of red blood cells

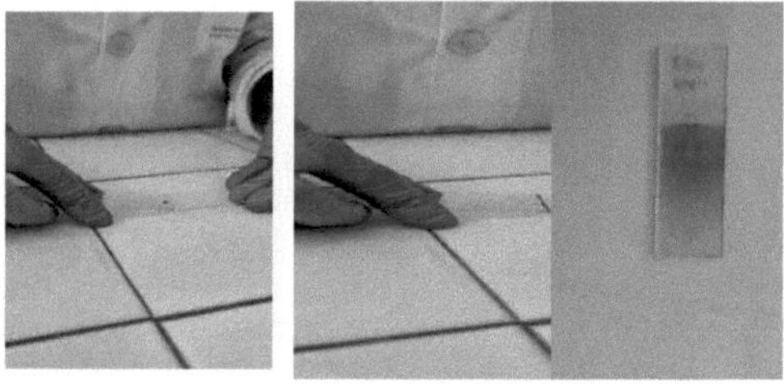

Figure 3: Preparation of a blood smear (HCN Parasitology Laboratory)

The smear is then fixed and stained with May Grünwald-Giemsa.Readings were taken at high magnification (x1000) for 20 minutes. i.e. a minimum of 200 fields to conclude that there are no parasites. The FS allows parasitised erythrocytes to be preserved, making it easier to diagnose the species, determine the stage of development and calculate the parasitaemia.

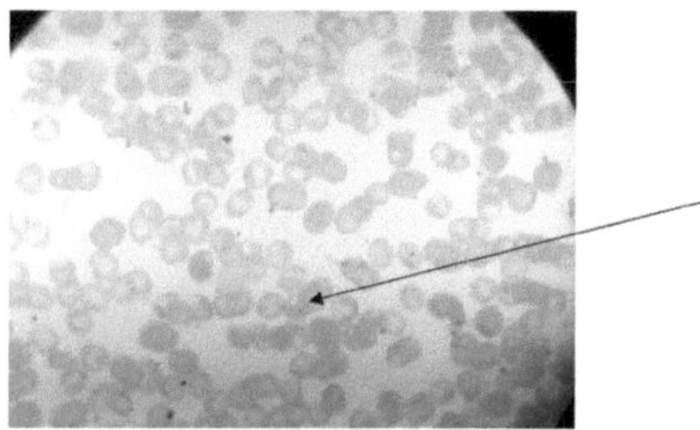

Figure 4: P. falciparum trophozoites on FS (MGG stain/ Obj x 100/ HCN parasitology laboratory)

- **Calculation of parasitaemia**

Parasitaemia was calculated as the average number of parasitised RBCs over 100 fields of the FS.

Number of parasitised red blood cells= Parasitaemia (in %) X100 Number of red blood cells in the field

2.4. Rapid diagnostic tests (RDTs) :

One, two or three rapid diagnostic tests (RDTs) were carried out on each sample, depending on availability in our laboratory.

The two main RDTs used in the laboratory during the study period were the "ABON™ Plus Malaria test®, Biopharm" and the "ABON™ Plus Malaria test". "iTest Malaria®, Bacterovir. The latter was introduced in 2021. Other tests were used when available, such as the "ONSite Pf/Pan Malaria®".

2.4.1 ABON Plus Malaria

a. Principle

This is an immunological test based on the principle of immunochromatography. It detects Plasmodium falciparum specific Histidine Richprotein (P.f HRP-2) antigens and aldolase, common to all 4 plasmodial species (P.f, Plasmodium malariae (P.m), Plasmodium vivax (P.v) and Plasmodium ovale (P.o)) in the whole blood of malaria patients. The membrane is coated with anti-P.f HRP-2 and anti-aldolase antibodies. During the test, the whole blood sample reacts with the coloured conjugate, which has been pre-coated on the test strip. The mixture migrates to the top of the membrane by capillary action and reacts with the anti-HRP2 antibodies on the membrane at the P.f test line and with the anti-aldolase antibodies on the membrane at the Pan line, leading to the formation of one or two coloured bands. The control band must always be coloured, otherwise the result is invalid.

b. Procedure

✓ Shake the blood tube before taking the test

✓ Transfer 10 µl of whole blood to well 1(W1) of the test device, then add 3 drops of buffer to well 2(W2).

✓ Start the stopwatch immediately.

✓ After 5 minutes, add 1 drop of buffer to W1

✓ The result should be read after 15 minutes.

c. Interpretation

➢P. falciparum infection: a line appears in the control region and a line in the P.f. region.

➢P. falciparum or mixed malaria infection: a line appears in the control region, a line in the Pan region and a line in the P.f. region.

➢Infection with P.non-falciparum: a line appears in the control region and a line in the Pan region.

➢Negative: a single line appears in the control region

➢Invalid: the line in the control zone does not appear.

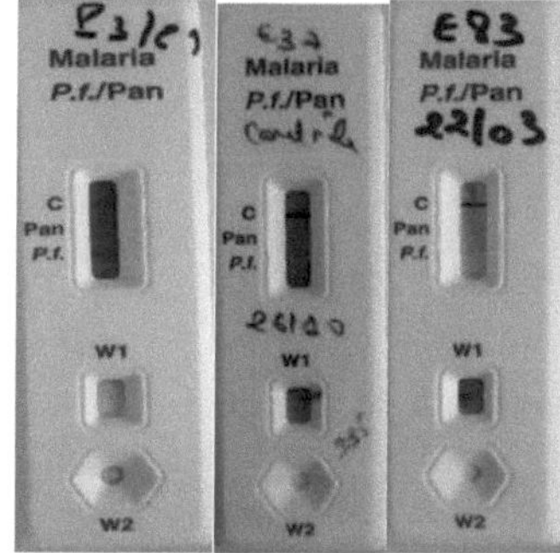

A b c

Figure 5: Different results of the ABON Plus Malaria test
a. positive test: P. falciparum infection

b. positive test: P. falciparum or mixed malaria infection

c. negative test

2.4.2 iTest®

a. Principle

The i test® casette is a qualitative membrane-based immunoassay for the detection of P. falciparum-specific HRP-2 antigen and pan-malarial aldolase antigen present in all four plasmodial species circulating in whole blood. The test uses a colloidal gold conjugate to selectively detect the antigens specific. During the test, and after the addition of the buffer, the blood sample migrates along the membrane and the colloidal gold particles conjugated with the anti-HPR2 and anti-aldolase antibodies will complex with the corresponding antigen. The complex migrates along the membrane where it is captured at the corresponding bands where the anti-HPR-2 and anti-aldolase monoclonal antibodies are coated, leading to the formation ofone or two coloured bands. The uncomplexed colloidal gold particles migrate along the membrane and are immobilised at the control band by a bound antibody. This control band is used to validate the test.

b. Procedure

✓ Place the case on a clean, flat surface

✓ Shake the blood tube before taking the test

✓ Draw 5 µL of whole blood using a pipette

✓ Add 3 drops of buffer

✓ Start the timer

✓ Read the results at 10 minutes

✓ Do not interpret results after 20 minutes

c. Interpretations

➢Positive: two or three lines of distinct colours

o P. falciparum infection and mixed malaria infection: one line in the C region, one line in the P.f region and one line in the Pan region.

o Infection with P. falciparum alone: one line in control C and one line in P.f.

o Infection by another species of P. non falciparum: one line in control C and one line in Pan.

➢Negative: a single line appears on the C control

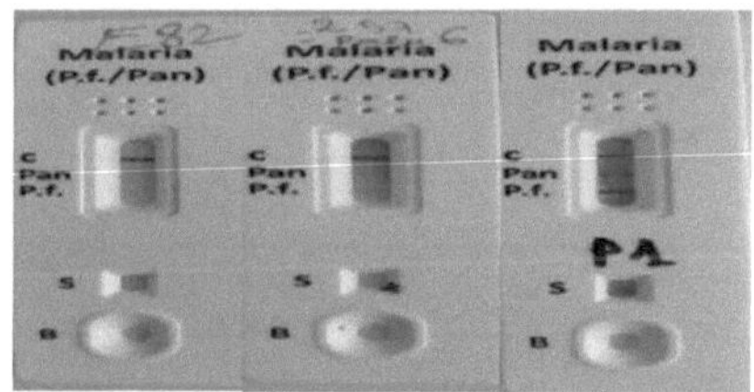

Non-valid : the line of control does not a b c

Figure 6: Different iTest® results

a. negative test

b. positive test: P. falciparum infection

c. positive test: P. falciparum or mixed malaria infection

IV. Reporting positive cases

All parasitic patients were notified by filling in the notification form for notifiable transmissible diseases on the register provided by the basic health care department. All these parasitic patients were then referred by the Department of School and University Medicine to the Infectious Diseases Department for treatment and follow-up.

V. Study statistics

The data were entered and processed using SPSS 21.0 software. For rapid diagnostic techniques, we calculated sensitivity, specificity, positive predictive value and negative predictive value. Agreement with the reference technique, which was the thick drop, was assessed by calculating Cohen's Kappa non-parametric test (Table I) and the observed agreement.

Table I: Interpretation of the Kappa concordance index

Kappa indexDegree of concordance	
<0	Very bad
0.01-0,20	Bad
0,21-0,40	Mediocre
0,40-0,60	Moderate
0,60-0,80	Good
0,80-1.00	Excellent

V. Search bibliography

The bibliography of our work was established by consulting the main databases (Medline and Embase) as well as the archive of the Faculty of Medicine of Tunis.

Scientific search engines used :

-PubMed(https://www.ncbi.nlm.nih.gov/pubmed),

-Science direct (https://www.sciencedirect.com)

-Google Scholar(https://scholar.google.com),

The key words used were: imported malaria, Plasmodium, Tunisia, diagnosis, rapid diagnostic test

VI. Ethical considerations and conflicts of interest :

Our study was carried out for academic non-profit purposes.

-Data was collected anonymously.

patients and the confidentiality of their information.

-There was no conflict of interest.

RESULTS

The diagnosis of malaria was based on the presence of Plasmodium sp on GE and/or FS. During the study period, out of a total of 271 people examined at the Parasitology-Mycology laboratory of the HCN in Tunis, we recorded 35 cases of imported malaria, i.e. 12.91%. These patients were divided into two different groups:

- Symptomatic patients referred with clinical suspicion of malaria.
- ENRPT referred by the Department of School and University Medicine as part of the national surveillance programme for this population. All were asymptomatic at the time of sampling.

I. Overall description of patients with malaria

1. Breakdown by gender

The majority of infected subjects were male (62.9%), with a sex ratio of 1.69 (Figure 7).

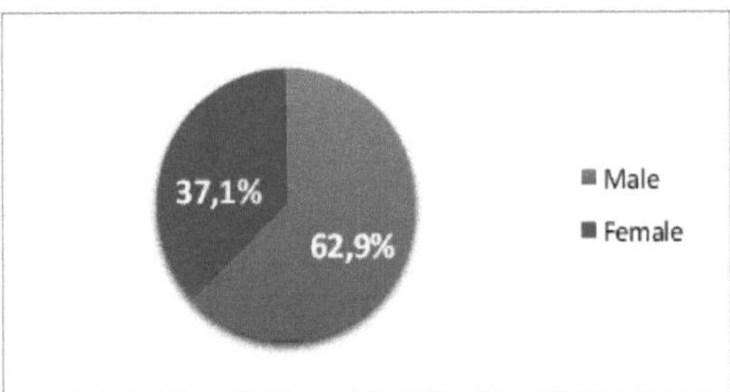

Figure 7: Breakdown of malaria cases by gender

2. Breakdown by age

The average age of infected patients was 26.7 ±8 years, with extremes ranging from 19 to 49 years. The age group most affected was between 20 and 24 (Figure 8).

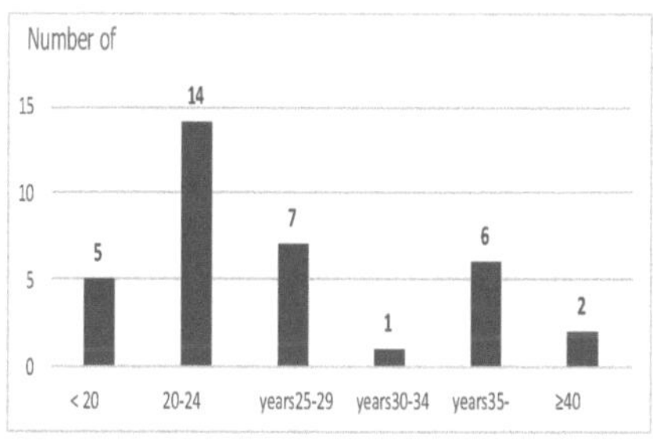

Figure 8: Breakdown of malaria cases by age

3. Annual distribution of cases of malaria

The maximum number of cases was recorded during the 2021-2022 academic year (n=21), i.e. 60% of all cases (Figure 9).

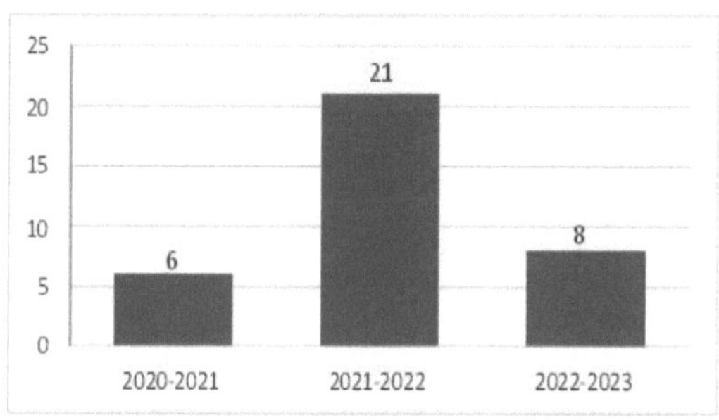

Figure 9: Annual breakdown of malaria cases

4. Presumed country of contamination

Sub-Saharan Africa was the origin of the majority of cases of contamination (94.3% of cases). The countries most affected were Côte d'Ivoire (20%) and Chad (14.3%) (Figure 10).

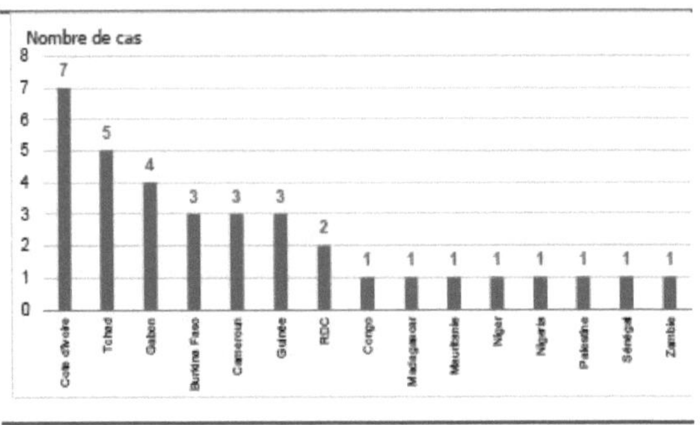

Figure 10: Breakdown by presumed country of infection

II. Epidemiological data according to the populations studied

1. Subjects symptomatic

Twenty-five patients were referred to our laboratory with symptoms suggestive of malaria. The majority (64%) came from various hospital departments, while the remainder (36%) were referred from the private sector (clinics).

Malaria was diagnosed in 12 of these patients, 5 of whom were Tunisians.

1.1. Breakdown by gender and age

The patients were predominantly male, with a sex ratio of 2. The mean age was 35, with extremes ranging from 23 to 49 years (Figure 11).

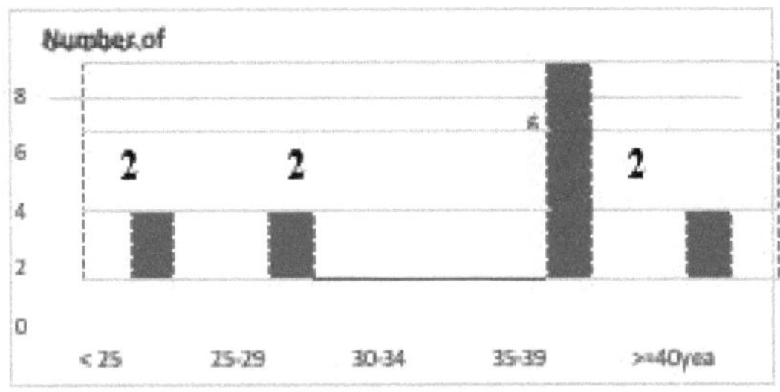

Figure 11: Age distribution of symptomatic patients

1.2. Breakdown by presumed country of contamination

All symptomatic patients were either from (n=7) or had stayed in sub-Saharan Africa (n=5). The most common country of origin was Côte d'Ivoire (5 cases), followed by Chad (3 cases) (Figure 12).

Tunisian patients (n=5):

- Three had spent time in Côte d'Ivoire
- A patient travelled between Côte d'Ivoire and Mali
- One patient had spent time in Burkina Faso

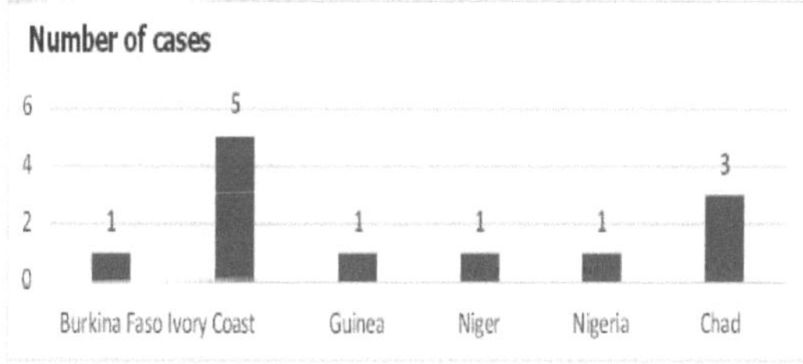

Figure 12: Breakdown of symptomatic cases by presumed country of infection

1.3. Chemoprophylaxis

None of the 5 infected Tunisian patients received antimalarial chemoprophylaxis during their stay in the malarious country.

1.4. Medical history of malaria

Only three of our patients reported at least one episode of malaria in their history, and two of these were Tunisians.

2. Asymptomatic subjects (ENRPT)

During the study period, which corresponded to three academic years, 246 ENRPT were screened in our laboratory. Asymptomatic carriage of Plasmodium was detected in 23 people, i.e. 9.35% of all students. The maximum number of cases was recorded in the 2021-2022 academic year (n=15) (Figure 13).

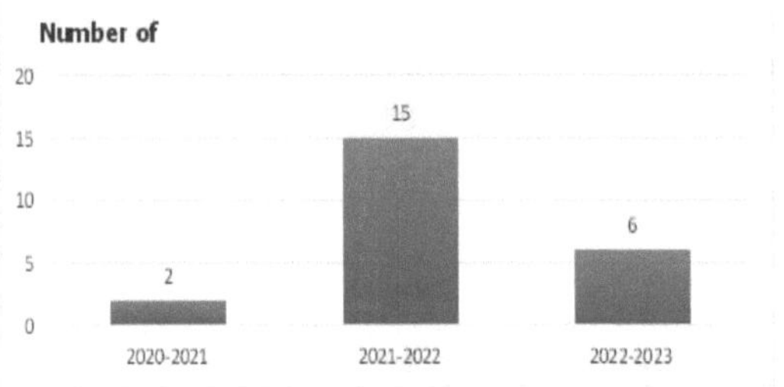

Figure 13: Annual distribution of infected ENRPTs

2.1. Breakdown by age and gender

A slight male predominance was noted among the infected students (n=13), with a sex ratio of 1.3. Their average age was 22.35±4 years, with extremes ranging from 19 to 33 years (Figure 14).

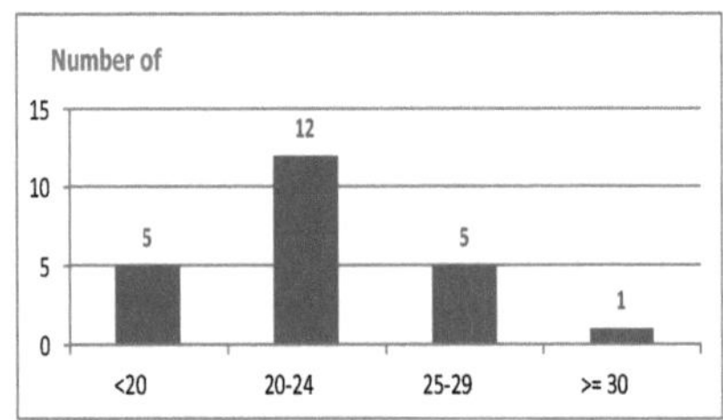

Figure 14: Age distribution of infected ENRPTs

2.2. Breakdown by origin geographical

Sub-Saharan Africa was the origin of the majority of parasitized ENRPT (91.3%). (Table II)

Table II: Distribution of parasitized students by geographical origin

Origin	Number
Sub-Saharan Africa	21
Maghreb	1
Middle East	1
Total	23

The most represented sub-Saharan African country was Gabon (n=4) followed by Cameroon (n=3) (Figure 15).

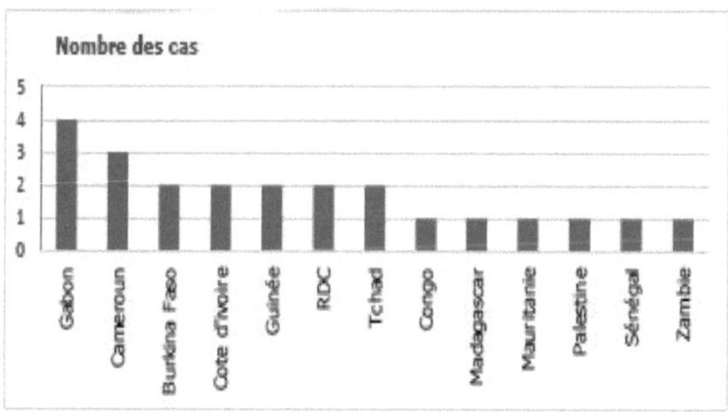

Figure 15: Breakdown of infected students by country of origin

2.3. Medical history of malaria

Ten of the 23 ENRPTs infected said they had contracted malaria at least once in their lives.

III. Results parasitological

1. Microscopy results (GE and FS)

- The diagnosis of malaria was based on a positive GE in 34 cases.
- The blood smear was positive in only 21 patients (11/12 symptomatic and 10/23 ENRPT), giving a sensitivity of 61.8% compared with GE.
- The last case was selected on the basis of two positive RDTs, even though the

microscopy did not reveal any Plasmodium: it involved a patient presenting with a fever on her return from a malaria zone and who had been self-medicated with Artemether-Lumefantrine prior to the consultation.

- The plasmodial species was identified on FS (n=21). The species most frequently identified was P. falciparum (20/21) (Figure 16).

A mixed infection was found in 3 cases, i.e. :

➢ P. falciparum + P. vivax association: 2 cases

➢ P. falciparum + P. ovale association: 1 case

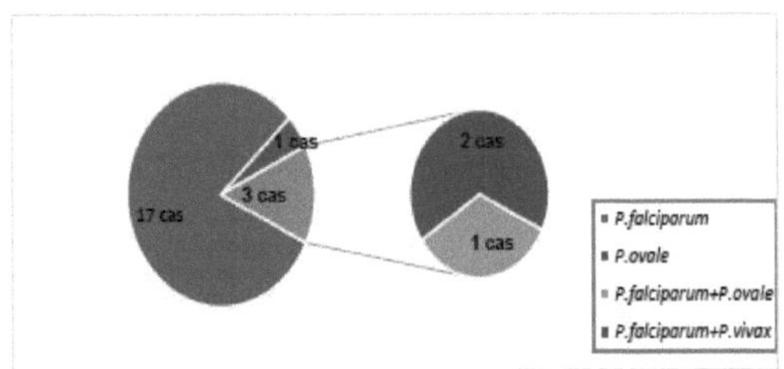

Figure 16: Breakdown of cases by plasmodium species

- The parasite stage was specified in 21 cases. The stages observed were :

➢ Trophozoites in 21 cases

➢ Gametocytes in 4 patients (2 cases of isolated P. falciparum, 1 case of P. ovale + P. falciparum and 1 case of P. vivax + P. falciparum)

➢ Schizonts in only 1 patient (P.vivax)

- In all asymptomatic cases (ENRPT), parasitaemia was very low (<0.1%). In symptomatic patients, it ranged from 0.5% to 20%, with a mean of 4.7% and a median of 3% (Tables IX and X).

2. Results of rapid diagnostic tests (RDT)

- All subjects referred to our laboratory (n=271) received at least one RDT in addition to microscopic investigation (FS+GE):

➤ The "ABON™ Plus Malaria" test® was carried out on almost all of these subjects (n=269).

➤ The "iTest Malaria" test® was introduced in 2021 and has been carried out on 176 people. Prior to its introduction, other tests were used depending on availability, such as the ONSite Pf/Pan Malaria® .

-Of the 34 cases diagnosed by microscopy, 67.6% (n=23) had at least one positive RDT and 26.5% (n=9) had 2 or more positive RDTs.

2.1. Results of RDT in symptomatic patients

- RDTs were positive in 10 of the 11 patients diagnosed by EW, giving a sensitivity of 91% (Table III).

- In addition, only one subject had 2 positive RDTs, although microscopy did not reveal any Plasmodium. This was a patient who presented with a fever after returning from a malaria zone and who had been self-medicated with Artemether-Lumefantrine prior to the consultation.

Table III: Results of RDTs (all types combined) in symptomatic subjects

	GE (+)	GE (-)	Total
TDR (+)	10	1	11
TDR (-)	1	13	14
Total	11	14	25

Using GE as the reference technique, the kappa coefficient showed an excellent concordance of 0.83 in symptomatic subjects, with an observed concordance of 92%.

2.1.1. Test "ABON™ Plus Malaria ® "

This test was performed in 23 of all symptomatic subjects referred to the laboratory, revealing 3 bands (C, Pan and P.f) in 4 cases and 2 bands (C and P.f) in 7 cases (table IV).

Table IV: Results of the ABON Plus® test in symptomatic subjects

	GE (+)	GE (-)	Total
ABON (+)	10	1	11
ABON (-)	0	12	12
Total	10	13	23

The sensitivity, specificity, positive predictive value (PPV) and negative predictive value (NPV) of this test compared with the GE used as the reference technique were 100%, 92%, 90% and 100% respectively. The observed concordance was 95.6% and the K coefficient was 0.91, showing excellent concordance between ABON Plus and GE in symptomatic patients.

2.1.2. iTest Malaria test ®

This test was introduced in our laboratory during the 2021-2022 academic year and was performed in only 10 of the symptomatic subjects. It came back positive in 3, revealing 3 bands in 1 patient and 2 bands in 2 others (Table V). Cohen's coefficient showed excellent agreement between the iTest® test and the GE (K=1).

Table V: Results of the iTest® test in symptomatic subjects

	GE (+)	GE (-)	Total
iTest (+)	3	0	3
iTest(-)	0	7	7
Total	3	7	10

2.2.Results of RDTs in asymptomatic subjects (ENRPT)

A total of 246 ENRPT had at least one RDT. Of the 23 ENRPT infected and diagnosed by microscopy (GE+), 13 had positive RDTs (Table VI).

Table VI: Results of RDTs (all types combined) in ENRPTs

	GE (+)	GE (-)	Total
TDR (+)	13	0	13
TDR (-)	10	223	233
Total	23	223	246

Using GE as the reference technique, the sensitivity, specificity, positive predictive value (PPV) and negative predictive value (NPV) were 56.5%, 100%, 100% and 95.7% respectively. The K coefficient was a good 0.7 and the concordance observed was 96% in asymptomatic subjects.

2.2.1. Test "ABON™ Plus Malaria ® "

This test was carried out on all 246 ENRPT screened. It came back positive in 11 individuals, revealing 3 bands in 7 cases and 2 bands in 4 cases (table VII).

Table VII: Results of the "ABON™ Plus Malaria®" test in ENRPTs

	GE (+)	GE (-)	Total
ABON (+)	11	0	11
ABON (-)	12	223	235
Total	23	223	246

Its sensitivity in relation to GE in asymptomatic subjects was 48% and its specificity was 100%. The PPV and NPV were 100% and 95% respectively.

The concordance observed was 95.1% and Cohen's Coefficient was a good 0.62.

2.2.2. iTest Malaria test ®

Since its introduction, 166 ENRPT have benefited from this test. Of these, 21 cases were diagnosed as having parasites by microscopy (GE+), although the test was positive in only 5 of them, showing 2 bands in 3 cases and 3 bands in 2 cases (table VIII).

Table VIII: Results of the "iTest Malaria®" test in ENRPTs

	GE (+)	GE (-)	Total
iTest (+)	5	0	5
iTest (-)	16	145	161
Total	21	145	166

The sensitivity, specificity, PPV and NPV of this test compared with the reference technique (GE) were 23.8%, 100%, 100% and 90% respectively. The kappa coefficient was a poor 0.35 and the agreement observed was 90.3%.

Table IX: Summary of parasitological data for symptomatic cases

Patient	GE	FS	Plasmodium species	Parasitic stage	Parasitaemia	ABON®Plus	iTest®	Other TDR
1	+	+	P. oval	Trophozoites	1%	NF	NF	OnSite -
2	+	+	P.f + P.o	Trophozoites (P.f+P.o) Gametocytes(P.f +P.o)	20%	+ (3 bands)	NF	NF
3	+	+	P.f + P. v	Trophozoites (P. f+P.v)	3%	+ (3 bands)	NF	OnSite +
4	+	+	P.f+ P.v	Trophozoites (P.f+P.v) Gametocytes(P.f +P.v)Schizontes (P.v)	2%	+ (3 bands)	NF	OnSite +
5	+	+	P. fTrophozoites Gametocytes		4%	+ (2 strips)	NF	OnSite +
6	+	+	P.f Trophozoites		3%	+ (2 strips)	NF	OnSite +
7	-	-	-	-	-	+ (2 strips)	NF	OnSite +
8	+	+	P.f Trophozoites		3%	+ (2 strips)	NF	NF
9	+	+	P.f Trophozoites		1%	+ (2 strips)	+ (2b)	OnSite +
10	+	+	P.f Trophozoites		0,5%	+ (2 strips)	NF	NF
11	+	+	P.f Trophozoites		2%	+ (3 bands)	+ (3b)	NF
12	+	+	P.fTrophozoites		12%	+ (2 strips)	+ (2b)	NF

NF: not done , P.f: Plasmodium falciparum,P.o: Plasmodium ovale,P.v: Plasmodium vivax

Table X: Summary of parasitological data from ENRPTs

GE		FS	ABON® plus	I TEST®
Patient 1	+	Gametocytes+trophozoites of P. f Parasitaemia< 1%	+ (3 bands)	NF
Patient 2	+	Trophozoites of P. f (Parasitaemia <0.1%)	+ (3 bands)	NF
Patient 3	+	-	-	-
Patient 4	+	-	-	-
Patient 5	+	-	-	-
Patient 6	+	Trophozoites of P.f (Parasitaemia <0.1%)	+ (3 bands)	-
Patient 7	+	+	+ Band P. f	-
Patient 8	+	-	-	-
Patient 9	+	-	-	-
Patient 10	+	-	+ (Weak band)	-
Patient 11	+	Trophozoites of P.f (Parasitaemia <0.1%)	+ (3 bands)	-
Patient 12	+	P. f trophozoites (parasitaemia<0.1%)	+ Band P. f	-
Patient 13	+	-	-	-
Patient 14	+	P. f trophozoites (parasitaemia<0.1%)	+	-
Patient 15	+	P. f trophozoites (parasitaemia<0.1%)	+ Band P. f	+ Band P. f
Patient 16	+	-	-	+ (3 bands)
Patient 17	+	-	-	+ P.f band
Patient 18	+	-	-	-
Patient 19	+	P. f trophozoites (parasitaemia<0.1%)	+ P.f band	+ P.f band
Patient 21	+	-	-	-
Patient 22	+	P. f trophozoites (parasitaemia<0.1%)	-	-
Patient 23	+	P. f trophozoites (parasitaemia<0.1%)	+ P.f band	+ P.f band

DISCUSSION

In view of the emergence of imported malaria in Tunisia, ongoing entomological and epidemiological surveillance is required in order to counter the risk of reintroduction of the parasitosis, which is constantly increasing with the intensification of international trade with malaria-infected countries, particularly in sub-Saharan Africa. In order to better define the parasitosis, it is essential to fine-tune certain techniques used in the biological diagnosis of malaria. It is in this context that our study was carried out, with the aim of evaluating the performance of two rapid diagnostic tests, ABON™ Plus Malaria® and iTest Malaria® , compared with the reference microscopic techniques (GE and FS), in the diagnosis of imported malaria in travellers to endemic areas and in the screening of students who are not permanent residents of Tunisia (ENRPT).

I. Main results

During the three academic years of our study (2020-2023), we received 271 consultants who were tested for parasitosis. Malaria was diagnosed in 35 cases. These positive cases were divided into 23 asymptomatic subjects diagnosed during systematic screening of ENRPT at the time of their enrolment in the various Tunisian institutions and 12 symptomatic subjects referred to our laboratory for clinical suspicion of malaria, 5 of whom were Tunisian nationals.

The majority of our cases were natives of or had lived in sub-Saharan Africa (94.3%). We noted a predominance of males among the infested subjects (63%) with a sex ratio equal to 1.69. The mean age was 26.7 years [19-49], with a predominance of cases in the 35-39 age group among symptomatic subjects and in the 20-24 age group among asymptomatic subjects. All subjects underwent an EWG, an FS and at least one RDT. 35 individuals were diagnosed as having malaria. Microscopy (a positive EWG) led to a positive diagnosis in 34 cases (97.14% of cases), while in the last case, the diagnosis was made on the basis of two positive tests, even though microscopy was negative, in a patient who had been self-medicated with antimalarial drugs prior to the consultation. The FS was positive in only 21 patients, i.e. a sensitivity of 61.8% compared with the GE considered as the reference technique. P. falciparum was the most commonly identified plasmodial species (95.23%). Parasitemia varied between the two study populations. It was very low in asymptomatic students diagnosed through screening (<0.1%) and varied between 0.5% and 20% in symptomatic patients. Regarding RDTs, we focused on the two tests that were in use in our laboratory during the study period. The ABON™ Plus test was performed in almost all individuals tested (n=269). The iTest® , introduced in 2021, was performed in only 176 individuals. Of the cases diagnosed by microscopy (GE+), 76.6% (n=23) had at least 1 positive RDT and 9 had 2 positive RDTs. Both tests showed excellent concordance with GE in symptomatic subjects with a K coefficient equal to 0.91 for the ABON™ Plus test and 1 for the iTest® .In asymptomatic students, the sensitivity, specificity, positive predictive value and negative predictive value of the ABON™ Plus test were 48%, 100%, 100% and 95% respectively and those of the iTest® were 23.8%, 100%, 100% and 90% and their concordance with GE was good (k=0.62) for the first test and poor (k=0.35) for the second.

II. Epidemiological data

Malaria is the most widespread parasitic disease in the world. It continues to rank among the top ten causes of death in low-income countries. In 2019, half of the world's population was at risk of malaria. contract the disease. According to the latest report on malaria in the world in 2023, it is estimated that there will be 5 million more cases of malaria in 2022 than in 2021 (249 million compared with 244 million). The WHO African Region alone was responsible for 94% of these cases (233 million cases). This increase can be explained by the disruption to malaria control services during the COVID-19 pandemic [2]. There has also been an increase in the number of deaths: an estimated 55,000 more people died from malaria in 2020 than in 2019 (631,000 compared with 576,000). However, the estimated number of deaths fell to 608,000 in 2022[2]. In Tunisia, the national malaria eradication programme was implemented in 1966. It comprised 4 phases: an attack phase (1967-1972), a consolidation phase (1973-1977), a maintenance phase (1978-1995) and a phase to prevent the reintroduction of malaria since 1996 [5]. It led to the elimination of malaria in 1979, the date of the last indigenous case, making our country the second country in the Maghreb to eliminate malaria after Libya [5,7]. Since then, another form of the disease has become established: imported malaria, the annual incidence of which is rising, although it is underestimated because of under-reporting, self-medication and cases that escape detection (illegal travellers, etc.). The annual incidence of cases has risen from less than ten cases in 1980 to more than 60 cases per year after 2010 [5,8](Figure 17).

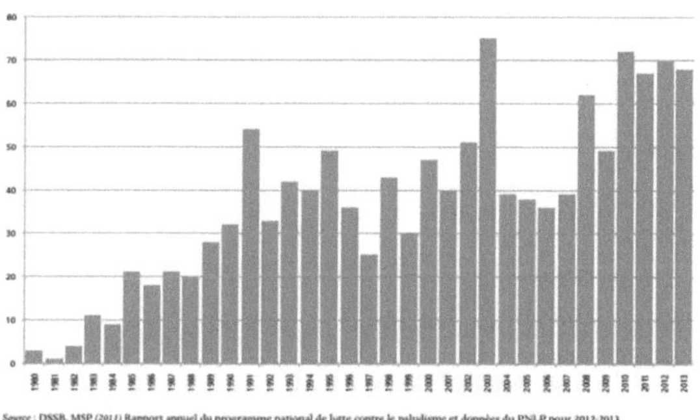

Figure 17: Number of imported cases recorded each year between 1980 and 2013 [8].

This increase is explained by the intensification of economic, commercial and professional exchanges with sub-Saharan Africa, especially with the recent introduction of direct flights between Tunisia and certain African capitals, and by the growing number of African students coming to Tunisia to pursue their higher education. These students, once infected with Plasmodium sp, constitute a potential reservoir of the parasite and, because of the persistence of anophelism, represent a risk of renewed transmission of this parasitosis. This has prompted increased vigilance against the disease and the maintenance of the prevention phase introduced in 1996, the main pillars of which are early treatment of new cases, compulsory reporting and ongoing entomological surveillance, as well as systematic active screening of ENRPTs. This last measure was introduced systematically in 1984 and is supervised in each university by the branches of the Department of School and University Medicine of the Ministry of Public Health. Every year, all foreign students are referred for screening before they leave the country. They should be referred to their local health laboratory or university hospital (CHU) for blood tests to detect malaria [9]. Our study identified 35 cases of malaria among 271 samples taken from symptomatic patients (12/25 positive cases) and ENRPT patients (23/246 positive cases) during screening, giving an overall prevalence of 13% (9.35% among ENRPT patients and 48% among symptomatic patients). In the Tunisian study carried out in the Parasitology-Mycology Department of La Rabta Hospital over a period of 17 years (1990-2006), involving 3476 ENRPT who had been screened for malaria, 128 were positive (i.e. 3.68%) [9]. In another study conducted by the same team in 2011, 3% of ENRPT were parasite carriers (3 cases/100 subjects tested) [10]. A more exhaustive study carried out over a 22-year period (1991-2012) identified 171 ENRPT with parasites [11].

Retrospective work carried out at the parasitology laboratory of the Institut Pasteur de Tunis (IPT) between January 2008 and September 2016 identified 85 cases of imported malaria, fourteen of which were asymptomatic cases detected during a systematic check of ENRPTs [12]. And in a thesis carried out in the same laboratory over a period of 25 months (2010-2012), Foudhaili et al noted an overall positivity rate of 12% (60/500 positive cases), with positivity rates of 22.9% in symptomatic subjects with clinical signs suggestive of malaria and 5 .2% during screening of asymptomatic ENRPT (16 positive cases out of 308 subjects tested) [13]. In a previous study by Aoun et al (199-2006), only 42 cases (1.7%) were recorded in 2478 asymptomatic subjects (ENRPT, immigrant workers from malaria-infected countries and Tunisians returning from endemic areas) sampled as part of the national malaria control programme with a view to systematic screening for malaria parasite carriage [14]. A comparison of the results of these different studies shows an increase over the years in the frequency of positive results for imported malaria, the highest being in our study (13%).The annual change in the number of cases showed a higher number in 2021-2022, corresponding to more than 3 times the number recorded in 2020-2021, then a decrease in 2022-2023, while remaining higher than in 2020-2021. This significant difference can be explained by the COVID-19 pandemic. The very low numbers in 2020-2021 are thought to be due to restrictions on movements and the closure of borders as a result of the pandemic, thus preventing ENRPTs from returning to their countries of origin during the holidays. Conversely, the very high figure for the following academic year could be explained partly by the resumption of air travel and the opening of borders, but also by the impact of the COVID 19 pandemic on the incidence of malaria in the African region. According to the 2021 WHO report, African areas with moderate to high malaria transmission experienced disruptions in malaria prevention, diagnosis and treatment services during the pandemic. As a result, between 2019 and 2020, the total number of malaria cases increased from 213 million to 228 million; the incidence of the disease rose from 222.9 to 232.8 cases per 1,000 inhabitants at risk of malaria, and the total number of deaths due to malaria rose from 534,000 to 602,000, with the mortality rate rising from 56 to 61.5 deaths per 100,000 inhabitants at risk of malaria [15]. A study of the demographic data of our patients showed a predominance of males (63% of cases). This predominance, which was even more marked in symptomatic patients (sex ratio =2), has been reported in all studies of imported malaria in Tunisia and worldwide [6,16-19].Men were more affected by malaria than women, which is This is probably due to the fact that men tend to travel abroad to study, and are also more exposed to mosquito bites in their home countries in connection with their activities [20].The average age of our patients was 26.7 years, with extremes ranging from 19 to 49 years. For symptomatic patients, the age group most affected was between 35-39 years, whereas for asymptomatic students, it was between 20-24 years. These results are similar to previous Tunisian studies reporting a predominance of cases diagnosed in young adults [8, 11, 12, 16].With regard to the presumed country of infection and geographical origin of patients, 85.7% of cases were foreigners and 14.3% were Tunisians (n=5). The latter accounted for 41.6% (5/12) of symptomatic patients. Sub-Saharan Africa was the main region involved (94.3% of cases), which is consistent with national data [8]. The most common country was Côte d'Ivoire (20% of cases), followed by Chad (14.3%). In Tunisia, as elsewhere in the world, various studies have identified West Africa as the primary source of infection. According to the study carried out by the Rabta team, 76.64% of cases came from this region, with the Ivory Coast the main country of infection (16.52% of cases), followed by Mali (14.9%) [11]. Results from the Institut Pasteur de Tunis (IPT) also highlighted the predominance of West African countries, with 29% of cases coming from the Ivory Coast [12]. This distribution correlates with the findings of the WHO report, which noted that in 2020, only six sub-Saharan African countries accounted for 55% of cases worldwide [15].

We looked for evidence of chemoprophylaxis in Tunisian subjects. Of the 5 patients with parasites, none had received chemoprophylaxis. This reluctance to take prophylactic medication has been noted in several Tunisian studies [11,17,21,22]. This non-compliance with chemoprophylaxis is thought to be This is primarily due to a lack of information and awareness among travellers about the seriousness of the parasitosis and the importance of prophylaxis against severe forms, but also to poor compliance with treatment secondary to poor tolerance and adverse effects of the drugs used. Information must be comprehensible and personalised for all travellers to endemic regions.

Recommendations must be clear and precise on the risks of infection and on preventive measures, including drug prophylaxis and personal protection against mosquito bites, which is often neglected by travellers [13].

III. Parasitological data

Malaria is a diagnostic and therapeutic emergency, given the unpredictable risk of rapid progression to the severe form. Diagnosis is essentially direct parasitological. According to WHO recommendations, parasitological confirmation must be obtained within less than two hours in order not to delay treatment. Microscopic examination of the thick blood drop and blood smear remain the gold standard in terms of sensitivity and specificity, and should be used as the first line of defence. They can be used to confirm the disease, identify the plasmodial species involved and assess parasitaemia, which has a bearing on both prognosis and treatment. However, the reliability of these tests requires equipment (microscope), quality reagents (dyes), a source of electricity and, above all, qualified personnel to carry them out [23]. All these factors have led to the development of RDTs (immunochromatographic tests) for the detection of parasitic antigens. They are currently used in association with microscopy. The advantage of these tests is that they are rapid and easy to use, making it possible to orientate or even confirm the diagnosis and to speed up treatment when access to microscopic examination proves impossible, especially in endemic areas [8].

1. Microscopy results

- Thick drop

EW is an enrichment technique based on microconcentration of the parasite. The parasites are released after lysis of the red blood cells. It offers very good sensitivity, even when parasitaemia is low, with a detection threshold of 10 parasites per microlitre (approximately 0.0002 to 0.0004%) [23,24,25].

One of the limitations of this excellent technique, apart from the need for the biologist to be experienced in reading it, is that it also depends on the quality of the microscope, the staining and the preparation technique. In addition, unlike FS, identification of plasmodial species and calculation of parasitaemia are difficult with EW. In our study, 34/35 cases were diagnosed as positive by EW and this method was considered to be the reference method on which the performance of the other parasitological diagnostic methods (FS and RDT) was based.

- Blood smear

FS has the advantage of preserving the morphological characteristics of Plasmodium and parasitized red blood cells (absence of haemolysis), thus allowing determination of the species and the stage of development of the parasite, as well as calculation of the parasitaemia, which has prognostic value and is useful for post-therapeutic monitoring [24]. However, this test is less sensitive than EW, with a detection threshold of 100 to 200 parasites per microlitre, which limits its performance for low parasitaemia levels, which is why it should always be combined with EW [26-28].

Of the 34 cases diagnosed by a positive GE, the FS was positive in only 21 patients, giving an overall sensitivity of 61.8% compared with the GE. This sensitivity varied between the two study populations. In fact, only 10 of the 23 asymptomatic subjects had a positive FS (43.47%), which can be explained by the very low parasitaemia (<0.1%) in these subjects, given that they were Immune (pre-armed) patients in whom the parasitaemia is well below the detection threshold of the FS, which is of the order of 100 to 200 parasites per microlitre (approximately 0.002 to 0.004%) [25]. This limitation of the FS has been described in several publications, which suggest that its theoretical sensitivity is 20 to 30 times lower than that of the thick drop [29]. In addition, the FS was positive in all our symptomatic patients with a positive GE (11/11) and whose parasitemia calculation revealed a parasite load that varied from

0.5% to 20% with a median of 3%. Two Tunisian patients (new non-immune subjects) had a parasitaemia >4% (12% and 20%), which corresponds to one of the WHO severity indicators and has a poor prognostic value.The limitations of microscopic diagnosis of FS could also be related to the variation in parasite density depending on the type of sample taken. In a study comparing the parasite densities of capillary and venous blood in asymptomatic carriers, the parasite detection rate was significantly higher in capillary blood than in venous blood [25]. This could support the hypothesis of sequestration or deep migration of the parasites at the schizont stage in cases of infection with P.falciparum, the most widespread species in the world and the only one isolated from our 10 FS-positive PRNTs. Concerning the species involved, identification was made by the FS in 21 individuals. Plasmodium falciparum was the predominant species in 95.23% of cases. We also recorded a single P. ovale infection and 3 mixed infections, 2 of which associated P. falciparum and P. vivax. Our results are in line with the national data published in the national guide to the management of malaria in Tunisia, which reports that P. falciparum is responsible for 86.8% of cases, while P. vivax and P. ovale infections account for 10.2% of cases [8]. Although the proportions of species vary according to the origin of imported cases, the predominance of P. falciparum is frequently observed in different countries. regions of the world. Mace et al report that 69.8% of imported malaria cases in the United States are due to P. falciparum, followed by P. vivax (9.5%) [30]. With regard to the evolutionary stages of Plasmodium sp, trophozoites were observed in 21 patients, P. vivax schizonts in a single patient and gametocytes in 5 patients (2 cases of isolated P. falciparum, 1 case of P. ovale + P. falciparum and 1 case of P. vivax + P. falciparum). Determining the stage of the parasite is important in view of its therapeutic implications (combination of gametocytocidal treatment). According to Aoun et al, the coexistence of parasitized individuals, the persistence of anophelism and the possibility of the introduction of new vector species as a result of climate change represent a real risk of infection of the latter by plasmodial gametocytes and therefore of the initiation of autochthonous transmission and reintroduction of the disease [14]. Once again, this underlines the importance of screening for this parasite.

2. RDT results

RDTs were developed in the early 1990s in an attempt to remedy the shortcomings of the health system in terms of malaria diagnosis, especially in certain endemic countries where access to microscopic laboratory diagnostic techniques is a real challenge. In 2012, the WHO launched its T3 (Test, Treat, Track) strategy, which encouraged the use of RDTs to guide diagnosis before treatment is started. The aim was to improve the proportion of malaria cases diagnosed, strengthen the surveillance system and avoid over-prescribing antimalarial drugs [31,32].

However, these RDTs should be considered as an aid to diagnosis. None of these tests can measure parasitaemia. They should not replace conventional microscopic techniques. These are immunochromatographic tests capable of detecting various plasmodial proteins in an average of 10-20 minutes.

Up to 3 different proteins can typically be tested on a single strip. The test is performed on a capillary or venous whole blood sample. The whole blood deposited on the RDT is lysed by the addition of a lysis buffer, the composition of which is specific to the test. Many manufacturers produce RDTs for malaria: while the monoclonal antibodies are of the same origin, the manufacture of the tests (concentration, conjugate, quality of nitrocellulose) is unique to each. Their production method and composition vary according to the antigen(s) detected: test presentations also vary in terms of device (cassette, strip, reaction card), antigens detected (1 to 3) and revelation system (conjugate marking) [23].
The RDTs currently available detect 3 types of antigen specific for Plasmodium sp [33] :

➢ Histidine-rich protein 2 (HRP2): an antigen specific to P. falciparum. It can persist in the body for up to 3ème weeks after recovery.

➢ Plasmodium lactate dehydrogenase (pLDH): a pan-specific antigen for the 5 plasmodial species (P. falciparum, P. vivax, P. ovale, P. malariae, P. knowlesi) or specific for P. falciparum, or specific for P. malariae.

P. vivax. It disappears rapidly after treatment

➢ Aldolase:It disappears rapidly after treatment.

There are several types of RDT, depending on the number of specific Plasmodium sp antigens they detect. A test detects either a single type of antigen, or two or three different antigens. The latter are known as combo tests. The RDTs used at Charles Nicolle Hospital, during the study period were ABON™ PLUS+ and iTEST® . These tests are combined, detecting both the monoclonal anti-HRP-2 antibodies and anti-aldolase antibodies. All subjects underwent at least one RDT (depending on kit availability).Of the 34 cases diagnosed by EW, 67.6% had one positive RDT and 26.5% had two or more positive RDTs. In symptomatic patients, when the results of RDTs (all types combined) were compared with EW, their sensitivity was 91%, whereas in asymptomatic subjects diagnosed during screening, it was 56.5%. This difference in sensitivity between the two groups can be explained by the poorer performance of these tests in cases of low parasitaemia, given that the detection threshold for these tests exceeds 100 parasites/µL. This explains their good performance in our symptomatic patients with high parasitaemia and their poor sensitivity in ENRPT (asymptomatic) patients with a parasite load of well below 0.1%.The lack of sensitivity of these tests is acceptable for diagnosing malaria in endemic areas where malaria attacks are usually accompanied by high parasite densities. However, it limits their usefulness for epidemiological studies in asymptomatic populations and in populations where parasite densities are low [31], such as the ENRPT population, who often have low parasite levels. In addition to the parasite load, the sensitivity of RDTs depends on the antigen sought, the quality of manufacture, the plasmodial species, the parasites living in the blood, compliance with the operating procedure and the examiner's interpretation [33].With regard to the antigen sought, the detection threshold varies from one test to another and from one species to another. The detection threshold for the HRP2 protein (specific to P.falciparum) is around 100 parasites/µl. As for the detection of aldolase (pan-specific antigen of the 4 plasmodial species), its sensitivity is lower than HRP2 for P. falciparum infections and remains moderate for other species, between 40 and 60% [34]. For P. vivax, tests detecting aldolase appear to perform less well than those detecting pLDH. For P. ovale and P. malariae infections, the detection of pan-aldolase performs poorly, similar to that obtained with the detection of parasitic pLDH [35]. Unfortunately, few KITS detecting this protein have been manufactured and placed on the market, with a limited number of studies on their performance. The evolution of the detection of this protein under treatment has not been studied.

Antigènes détectés	Espèces plasmodiales détectées	Sensibilité
HRP2	*P. falciparum*	++++
Pf. pLDH	*P. falciparum*	+++
Pv. pLDH	*P. vivax*	+++
Pv. aldolase	*P. vivax*	++
Pan pLDH	*Plasmodium sp.*	-*
Pan aldolase	*Plasmodium sp.*	-*
* données pour la détection de *P. ovale* et de *P. malariae*.		

Figure 18: Relative sensitivity of rapid diagnostic tests according to the nature of the antigen detected [35].

In our study, there were 10 false-negative cases (in ENRPT with P. falciparum on FS with negative RDT). As mentioned above, this can be explained essentially by the low parasitaemia in this population, but could also be due to a deletion of the gene encoding HRP-2, or a decrease or variation in its expression

[36]. This hypothesis was the subject of various studies revealing genetic diversity in the HPR- 2 sequences of P. falciparum [37]. Thus, P. falciparum that does not express histidine-rich protein 2 (HRP2) may escape detection by RDTs based on HRP2 detection. In addition, histidine-rich protein 3 (HRP3), a homologous protein of HRP2, may cross-react with monoclonal antibodies used for HRP2 detection at densities of of parasites. P. falciparum parasites that express neither HRP2 nor HRP3 are completely undetectable by HRP2-based RDTs. According to data provided by manufacturers, approximately 415.5 million of these RDTs were sold in 2022. The WHO recommends that countries where PfHRP2/3 deletions have been reported, as well as neighbouring countries, conduct representative baseline surveys among suspected malaria cases to determine whether the prevalence of PfHRP2/3 deletions causing false-negative RDT results exceeds the threshold requiring a change of RDT[2].

Antigen production also varies between the evolutionary stages of the parasite; HRP2 predominates in the asexual and young gametocyte stages [37] whereas the other antigens are produced by the different sexual and asexual stages of the parasite. This could be another explanation for the false negatives in our study. Failure to comply with the conditions of use or incorrect interpretation of the tests by the operator could also lead to false negative or positive results. We also noted one case where the diagnosis was made retrospectively on the basis of two positive RDTs despite the negativity of the microscopy. This case involved a patient who had been self-medicated with Artemether-Lumefantrine for symptoms suggestive of malaria on her return from a malaria zone, before seeking medical advice. In fact, according to Brenier, HRP-2 RDTs can be useful for establishing a diagnosis a posteriori of a syndrome labelled malaria and treated before biological confirmation, because of the persistence of this antigen in the blood for weeks after recovery [38]. For the same reason, these RDTs are considered to be of little or no value in post-treatment follow-up [39].

2.1. Test "ABON™ Plus Malaria ® "

During the study period, this test was used in a total of 269 individuals, divided into 23 symptomatic patients with suspected malaria and 246 ENRPT asymptomatic patients tested as part of systematic screening. For symptomatic subjects, this test demonstrated good reliability with excellent concordance with the thick drop (reference technique) in the detection of malaria infections with a sensitivity of 100%, a specificity of 92% and positive and negative predictive values of 90% and 100% respectively. Our results were comparable to the values claimed by the manufacturer, i.e. a sensitivity of between 94.5% and 100% for P. falciparum and between 98.1% and 100% for the other species (the detection thresholds were not precise) and a specificity of between 97.3% and 99.8% [40]. Our results were close to those of other studies such as Djoba Siawaya et al, which showed a sensitivity of 91% and positive and negative predictive values of 99% and 98% [41]. Thus, according to our study, the performance of this test in this group of symptomatic subjects was in line with WHO recommendations, which require a minimum sensitivity of 95% for parasitaemia ≥100 parasites/μL [27]. This justifies the usefulness and effectiveness of this test in emergency departments to guide the management of suspected malaria cases, especially when access to a specialised laboratory is difficult.In addition, a study of the performance of this test in the population of asymptomatic students (screening framework) showed a lower sensitivity (48%) with a specificity, PPV and NPV of 100%, 100% and 95% respectively and a concordance coefficient K=0.62. This makes the test useful when positive, but unreliable (risk of false negatives) in detecting infections with low parasitaemia.

2.2. iTest Malaria test ®

This test was introduced during 2021-2022 and was carried out in 176 individuals, 10 of whom were malaria suspects and 166 of whom were asymptomatic students. According to the manufacturer, this test has a sensitivity for P. falciparum of between 96.5% and 100% for a detection threshold of 200 parasites/µL and a sensitivity for P.vivax of between 90.3% and 100% for a detection threshold of 1500 parasites/µL. The specificity of this test is 99.4% to 100% (Technical Data Sheet). In our study, in symptomatic subjects, this test had a sensitivity of 100% with excellent concordance with the GE (K=1), in line with the previous test. However, this was not the case with asymptomatic subjects in whom the iTest® showed a very low sensitivity of 23.8%, a specificity of 100%, a PPV of 100% and an NPV of 90%. Agreement with GE was poor (K coefficient = 0.35). Like the ABON Plus®, the iTest® meets WHO requirements for parasitaemia ≥100 p/µL and appears to be a reliable tool in symptomatic subjects, but its performance is much lower in screening asymptomatic subjects with low parasitaemia.Unfortunately, our results could not be compared with other studies. None of them looked at the evaluation of this new kit on the market.A comparison of the 2 RDTs reveals a difference in sensitivity in the ENRPT population, despite the fact that they are based on the same principle and detect the same antigens. This clearly shows that the source of antigen used to induce TDR antibodies (purified native protein, recombinant proteins, or peptides) could make significant differences in the performance characteristics of the test. Even monoclonal antibodies directed against the same antigen, if they target different epitopes of that antigen, can have very different sensitivities and specificities [36].

Limitations of the study :

- In the course of carrying out this work, we were confronted with certain limitations, such as :

✓ The lack of information on travel and means of antimalarial protection, which was not always available or detailed. Indeed, as with any retrospective study, missing data are difficult to retrieve. Similarly, no information was available on the follow-up of patients diagnosed with malaria, particularly post-treatment follow-up, since these patients are referred to other hospitals for further treatment.

✓ The second limitation was that the rapid diagnostic kits studied and used in our laboratory during the study period were based on the same principle and looked for the same antigens, making it difficult to compare and accurately study their performance.

✓ The difficulty in evaluating the iTest kit® lies in the lack of information and experience with this test, which has just been launched on the market in France.

Outlook:

- Our study showed that a significant number of cases of imported malaria were recorded among nationals of endemic countries outside the student population, which raises the question of extending the circle of systematic screening to people from sub-Saharan Africa.

-It should also be noted that chemoprophylaxis was neglected in Tunisian subjects, who accounted for almost half of our symptomatic cases. For this reason, it seems that additional efforts should be made to raise awareness and promote pre-travel consultations.

- As far as diagnostics are concerned, although rapid diagnostic tests have demonstrated their reliability in diagnosing symptomatic subjects, they have shown their limitations in the context of screening asymptomatic subjects. Similarly, microscopy (GE and FS), considered to be the "gold standard" in malaria diagnosis, has also shown its limitations due to the difficulty of reading it when parasitaemia is very low. Thus, the best performing and most effective alternative is PCR would be the most appropriate for screening purposes. It is a highly sensitive technique with a detection threshold of 0.3p/ml. It can also be used to diagnose species. Its usefulness has been well studied and detailed in the publication by Savary et al, which focused on travellers receiving chemoprophylaxis and having low parasitaemia levels. When carried out under the right conditions, PCR has been shown to have an excellent negative predictive value and specificity of 100% [42].

However, its high cost, the need for specialised equipment and its relatively long turnaround time are obstacles to its routine use and to its availability in all laboratories (not available in our laboratory).

CONCLUSIONS

Malaria is a formidable global scourge for which the African continent continues to pay the heaviest price. The increase in the number of cases of imported malaria reported in Tunisia, which has been certified malaria-free, means that strict surveillance is needed and preventive measures must be stepped up to minimise the risk of its reintroduction into our country. This requires the introduction of a strategy for the rapid and effective diagnosis and treatment of exposed (symptomatic) individuals, and systematic screening of people from malaria-endemic areas. The aim of our work was to evaluate the performance of two rapid diagnostic tests ABON™ Plus Malaria® and iTest Malaria® compared with reference microscopic techniques, in the diagnosis of imported malaria in travellers to endemic areas and in screening non-permanent resident students in Tunisia (ENRPT). We conducted a descriptive, retrospective study of 35 cases diagnosed at the Parasitology-Mycology laboratory of Charles Nicolle Hospital in Tunis over a period of three academic years: 2020-2021/ 2021-2022 and 2022-2023. These patients were divided into two different groups: symptomatic subjects referred for clinical suspicion of malaria and ENRPT referred by the Directorate of School and University Medicine as part of the national surveillance programme for this population. Sub-Saharan Africa was the origin of the majority of our patients (94.3%). They were male in 63% of cases and their average age was 26.7 years, with extremes ranging from 19 to 49 years. Parasitological diagnosis was based on EW, FS and at least one RDT in all subjects (ENRPT and patients). In order to study the performance of the diagnostic techniques, EW was considered to be the reference technique for its very high sensitivity. The FS enabled the plasmodial species to be identified in 21 cases. P. falciparum was the most commonly identified species, present in 20/21 cases, with 3 cases of mixed infection associating other plasmodial species: 2 associating P. vivax and 1 associating P. ovale. Parasitaemia, which was calculated on FS, varied between 0.5 and 20% in symptomatic patients, whereas it was very low in asymptomatic subjects (ENRPT) (<0.1%). With regard to rapid diagnostic tests, different kits were used in our patients (depending on availability). They had a combined sensitivity of 91% in symptomatic subjects and 56.5% in asymptomatic subjects. The low sensitivity described in the latter group is explained by the low parasitaemia in this population. It can therefore be concluded that RDTs are a useful diagnostic aid for the rapid management of symptomatic subjects with suspected malaria, but their performance is limited in cases of low parasitaemia, either during screening or in patients who have received chemoprophylaxis. They are therefore no substitute for conventional microscopic techniques. PCR would be a more effective alternative, better suited to screening and in situations where microscopic diagnosis is difficult. At the end of this study, the number of cases of imported malaria, which represent a potential reservoir of the parasite, remains significant. It is therefore important to continue screening at-risk populations and to stress to travellers the importance of pre-travel consultations and compliance with prophylactic measures.

REFERENCES

1.Argy N, Houzé S. Epidemiology and parasite cycle of a global scourge, malaria. Pharmaceutical News. Mar 2018;57(574):18-20.

2.World Health Organisation. World malaria report 2023. Available at URL: https: //www.who.int/teams/global-malaria-programme/reports/world- malaria-report-2023.

3.Chadli A, Kennou MF, Kooli J. Malaria in Tunisia: history and present status. Bull Soc PatholExot Filiales. 1985;78(5 Pt 2):844-51.

4.Chahed MK, Bouratbine A, Krida G, Ben Hamida A. Receptivity of the Tunisian to malaria afteritseradication:analysis of the situation for adequacy of the surveillance. Bull Soc PatholExot. 2001 Aug;94(3):271-6.

5.World Health Organisation. Eliminating malaria and preventing its recurrence in Tunisia: an exemplary success story. 1st edition. Geneva: World Health Organization. 2015; 6.

6.Bouratbine A, Chahed K, Aoun K, Krida G, Ayari S, Ben Ismail R. Imported malaria in Tunisia. Bulletin de la Société de pathologie exotique. Jan 1998; 91(3): 203-7.

7.Ba O, Ouldabdallahi M, Koïta M, Sy O, Dahdi SA. Epidemiology of malaria and elimination prospects in Maghreb Countries. Tunis Med. 2018 Oct-Nov;96(10-11):590-598.

8.Bouzouaya N. Guide National De Prise en Charge Du Paludisme En Tunisie. 2ième edition. Tunis: World Health Organization; 2016.

9.Sghaier L, Yaakoub A, Anene S et al. Blood and urinary parasitosis in non-permanent resident students in Tunisia. RevTunInfectiol2008;2:32-6.

10. Doctoral thesis in medicine. Aicha kallel. Diagnosis of malaria: comparative study of three techniques: thick drop and blood smear, test of rapid diagnosis and nested PCR. Faculty of Medicine of Tunis. defended on 19/11/201.

11. Dridi K, Fakhfakh N, Belhadj S, Kaouech E, Kallel K, Chaker E. Malaria in Tunisia: A propos of 432 cases diagnosed at the Chu La Rabta of Tunis (1991-2012). Revue tunisienne de biologie clinique. 2015;22(1):16-22.
12. Mtibaa L, Siala E, Bouhlel S, Abda IB, Abdallah RB, Zallega N, et al. Imported malaria in Tunisia: assessment of diagnostic cases at the Pasteur Institute of Tunis (2008-2016). Pan Afr Med J. 2017;4(4):34.
13. Doctoral thesis in medicine. Hela Foudhaili. Evaluation of the performance of the Optimal -IT® test in the diagnosis of imported malaria. Defended 27/0/2013
14. Aoun.k, Siala.E, Tchibkere.D, Ben Abdallah.R, Zallega.N, Chahed.MK, Bouratbine.A. Imported malaria in Tunisia: consequences on the risk of reintroduction of the disease.2010 ;70 :33-37.
15. World Health Organization. World Malaria Report 2021, Key messages WHO/UCN/GMP/2021.08.
16. Belhadj S, Menif O, Kaouech E, Anane S, Jeguirim H, Ben Chaabane T, et al. Imported malaria in Tunisia: review of 291 cases diagnosed at La Rabta Hospital in Tunis (1991-2006). RevFrancoph Lab. Fév2008;2008(399):95-8.
17. Bouchair A. Imported malaria in adults in Tunisia: a study of 190 cases [thesis: medicine]. Tunis: Tunis Faculty of Medicine; 2017.
18. Legros F. Imported malaria in France: surveillance methods and main epidemiological characteristics. Lettre Infect. 2008;13(3):100- 22.
19. Thellier M, Kendjo E, Houzé S, Bras JL, Danis M. Epidemiology of malaria worldwide: real hope for disease control, but new concerns. LettInfectiol. 2012;27(6): 216-21.
20. Kristina M. Angelo, Michael Libman ,EricCaumes , Davidson H. Hamer , Kevin C. Kain , Karin Leder, et al. Malaria after international travel:aGeo Sentinel analysis, 2003-2016. Malar J (2017) 16:293.
21. Chelaifa M, Mtibaa L, Abbes S, Besrour R, Ben aziza A, JemliB. Imported malaria in Tunisia: review of cases diagnosed at the Tunis Military Hospital

(2012-2020). STPI [Online]. 2021. Available at URL: https://www.infectiologie.org.tn/uploadEposter/4658.pdf
22. Dahmeni, A. Antimalarial chemoprophylaxis in cases of imported malaria [Dissertation: Travel medicine]. Tunis: Tunis Faculty of Medicine; 2019.
23. Houzé . Rapid Diagnostic Test for Malaria .Bull. Soc. Pathol. Exot. 2017;110:49-54.
24. Chaker.E. Le paludisme : Diagnostic parasitologique.2000 :1-4
25. Ouedraogo. Jb ,Guiguemde.Tr , Gbary .Ar. Comparative study of parasite densities from venous and capillary blood during malaria. 1991 ; 38(8/9) : 601-605.
26. Durieux MF. Biological diagnosis of malaria. Actual Pharm. Mar 2018;57(574):25-9.
27. De Gentile L, Geneviève F. Imported malaria: laboratory diagnosis. Revue Française des Laboratoires. Mar 2000;2000(321):25-9.
28. Siala E, Ben Abdallah R, Bouratbine A, Aoun K. Update on the biological diagnosis of malaria. RevTun Infect. 2010;4:5-9.
29. Association Française des Enseignants de Parasitologie et Mycologie. Malaria [Online]. ANOFEL [cited 6 Jan 2023]. Available from URL:https://fr.readkong.com/page/paludisme-association-francaise- des-enseignants-de-6695706.
30. Mace KE. Malaria Surveillance - United States, 2018. MMWR SurveillSumm [Online]. 2022 [cited 7 Jan 2023];71. Available from URL: https://www.cdc.gov/mmwr/volumes/71/ss/ss7108a1.html
31. Moody A. Rapid Diagnostic Tests for Malaria Parasites. Clin Microbiol Rev. Jan 2002;15(1):66-78.
32. World Health Organization. Test, treat, track: scaling up diagnostic testing, treatment and surveillance for malaria [Online]. World Health Organization; 2012 [cited 8 Jan 2023]. Available from URL: https://apps.who.int/iris/handle/10665/337979.

33. Munier A, Diallo A, Sokhna C, Chippaux JP. Evaluation of a rapid malaria diagnostic test in rural health posts in Senegal. Médecine Tropicale ; 69(5): 496-500, 2009.
34. Berry A, Iriart X, Magnaval JF. New methods for diagnosing malaria. Rev Francoph Lab. Nov 2009;2009(416):65-70.
35. De Carsalade.GY ,LamKam.R , Lepere .JF, De Brettes .A , Peyramond .D. Is it possible to replace the smear/thick drop test with a rapid diagnostic test for the diagnosis of malaria? L'expérience de Mayotte.2008; 39(2009) :36-40.
36. Clinton K. Murray, Robert A. Gasser Jr , Alan J. Magill, and R. Scott Miller. Update on Rapid Diagnostic Testing for Malaria.2008 ;21(n°1) : 97-110

37. Baker.J , McCarthy.J, Gatton.M, E Kyle.D, Belizario.V, Luchavez.J,.D, Cheng.Q. Genetic diversity of Plasmodium falciparum histidine-rich protein 2 (PfHRP2) and its effect on the performance of PfHRP2-based rapid diagnostic tests.2005 ;192(5) :870-7.
38. Brenier-Pinchart MP, Pinel C, Grillot R, Ambroise-Thomas P. Diagnosis of malaria in non-endemic regions: value, limitations and complementarity of current methods. Ann Biol Clin (Paris). 9 June 2000;58(3):310-6.

39. Mercier V, Bailly É, Langendonck N, Chevallier E, Bernard L, Desoubeaux G. Tricks and misuses of rapid diagnostic testing for malaria diagnosis. Ann Biol Clin (Paris). 2020;78(2):174-176
40. ABON Malaria P.f./Pan Rapid Test Device (Whole Blood) [online]. [cited 10 Jan 2023]. Available from URL: https://itama.co.id/wp-content/uploads/2021/11/1.-ABON-Malaria-IMA-T402-Brochure.pdf
41. Djoba Siawaya J. Evaluation of SdBioline Malaria ANTIGEN Pf/Pan (HRP2/pLDH). 2014.
42. Savary P. Advice to the pharmacy for the prevention of malaria in travellers, situation in 2018. Pharmaceutical Sciences. 2019.

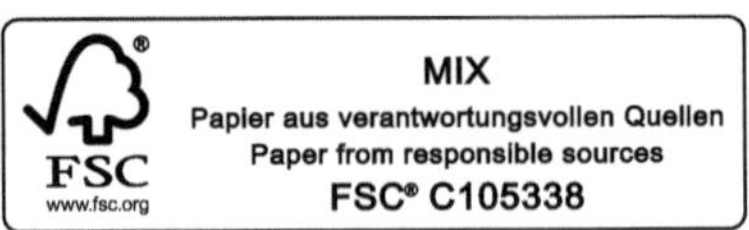

Printed by Books on Demand GmbH, Norderstedt / Germany